Muscle Building Guide for Beginners:

14 Essential Tips for Maximizing Muscular Growth

By Frantzky Jean

Copyright Page
Muscle-Building Guide for Beginners: 14 Essential Tips for Maximizing Muscular Growth

First Edition

Notable Quotes

"The first wealth is health." –Ralph Waldo Emerson

"Eighty percent of success is showing up." -Woody Allen

"If you always put limit on everything you do, it will spread into your work and into your life. There are no limits. There are only plateaus, and you must not stay there, you must go beyond them." –Bruce Lee

"Take care of your body. It's the only place you have to live." –Jim Rohn

Introduction

Whether it's jogging, sprinting, swimming, or walking - physical exercise is important for maintaining health, vitality and physiological well-being. There probably isn't a single doctor in the world who would discount the significance of daily physical activity to the human body. But what we all can agree on in terms of physical activity is that running, walking and jogging cannot facilitate the body's ability to produce lean muscle mass and strength. Here is where weightlifting often comes into play. Individuals who want to fulfill their fitness goals of building their muscular physique and becoming stronger than ever must apply some form of resistance training. Weightlifting is the ultimate form of resistance training and could help the body develop stronger, tougher and bigger muscles down the road. If done properly and persistently, intense resistance training could work wonders to your body composition and muscles.

However, what often bothers me is the fact that beginners who are relatively new to weightlifting never seem to have any clue about how to effectively build lean muscle mass and strength in an efficient manner. Beginners so often fail to realize that the decisions that they make outside the gym are just as important as the decisions they make inside the gym. Consequently, I find many beginners often struggling and becoming frustrated about their lack of success in obtaining their fitness goals. Some of them want to build muscle, others look for strength, and others value muscle growth, strength and size while burning fat. Regardless of what fitness goals you're trying to accomplish, I believe that these 14 tips that I'm about to share with you will help guide you to maximizing the productivity of your training routine and help you gain wisdom of how muscle-building works. These 14 essential tips will help accelerate the muscle growth process and facilitate gains in strength and size. Hopefully, you will see the underlying value of these simple tips and begin to implement them in your daily life. Enjoy!

Tip #1: Drink Plenty of Water

The vast majority of people already know that water is one of the few resources present on Earth that humans cannot live without; along with food, air and shelter. But what many of us may not know about water is that it helps stimulate muscle growth and development, enabling muscle builders to add on lean mass more efficiently. This is because the greatest portion of our bodies, approximately 60% of our total body weight, is composed of water. About seventy-five percent of our muscle tissue is made up of water! By being deprived of one of nature's most essential resources, you're causing havoc to the body, the muscle tissues and even the brain that's made up of 77% of, you guessed it, water!

Water consumption is probably one of the most overlooked aspects of dieting for men and women seeking to fulfill their goals to add lean muscle. On the opposite spectrum, savvy bodybuilders who acknowledge the significance of drinking water experience astounding results in addition to eating a clean, protein-rich diet. There has even been surprising reports of some bodybuilders drinking a total of nearly 10 liters of water daily! In order to maximize muscle growth and size, you must be willing to nourish the muscle tissues with what it's primarily comprised of. As Blake Bissaillion of Muscle-building 101 explains, "Water is the medium in which all energy reactions take place. Therefore, you need to drink a lot of water for health, stamina, fuel, and building muscle." No true bodybuilder or individual for that matter can't survive and thrive without the consumption of clean water.

Drinking enough water will also promote weight loss by making you feel full longer and serving as a replacement for obesity-ridden carbonated sodas, energy drinks, artificial juices, alcohol, etc. Not to mention the fact that more than one-third of U.S adults (34.9%) are already obese, according to the Centers for Disease Control and Prevention. Bottom line, consuming water is an absolute must for maintaining a healthy body and developing stronger and leaner muscles. Other notable benefits of water consumption are the elimination of toxins and waste products from the body, reduced chances of potential headaches and improved digestion.

So how much water should you consume? Some sources recommend you follow a general guideline of total fluid intake (including other beverages and food) of around 90 ounces per day for women and 120 ounces for men. Other sources recommend drinking a minimum of half your bodyweight in ounces of water. For example, if Tom weighs 180 pounds then it is recommended that he consumes at least 90 ounces of water every day. I recommend the "half-your-bodyweight" guideline as a rule-of-thumb. You can choose to follow one of these popular guidelines or create your own practical guideline, just make sure drinking plenty of water on a daily basis.

In closing, avoid drinking water from sources that are more exposed to high amounts of fluoride; such as tap water, community water (water fountains) and certain bottled brands with added fluoride. There are tons of reasons why it is necessary for you take every precaution to avoid consuming fluoridated water; primarily because it has been linked to bone fractures, thyroid disorders and impaired brain development and function. Opt for buying spring bottled water brands in the stores or try purchasing a reliable water filtration system, like the Propur Big with ProOne Filters from infowarsshop.com.

Summary: A large percentage of the body, brain and muscle tissues are all made up of water. If you want to gain maximum results in muscle growth, strength size, then consuming large amounts of water has to become a top priority in your daily life. A healthier brain, skin and digestive system are also great benefits of drinking clean water.

Tip #2: Maintain a Clean Diet

If you are one hundred percent committed to packing on pounds of muscles to your frame, then not fully acknowledging the significance of a healthy, well-balanced diet is nonsensical. This is because regardless of how much you train or lift, without a solid diet plan that incorporates nutritious calories, protein and fats essential for muscle growth, you can kiss your muscle-building goals good-bye. Just like how 2 plus 2 always equals 4, if you want to build muscle and gain healthy weight then you must consume more calories to facilitate the muscle-building process. That doesn't mean to start devouring any form of calories from foods like French fries, hamburgers, pizzas, baked goods, and sodas. These common foods are what I like to call hazardous and toxic to the health of the American public. These foods and many others are formally labeled as having "empty" calories because they do not offer any nutritional value to the body, brain and muscles. If you are serious about reaching your muscle-building potential and establishing a physique that boasts pure strength, then you must focus on implementing "quality" calories, proteins and fats into your diet. Foods like wild salmon and other fish products, whole eggs, chicken, turkey, mixed nuts, lean red meats, fruits and veggies are essential for any muscle-building plan. These foods not only boast high-quality calories and protein suitable for lean muscle mass, but foods like wild salmon and tuna are incredible sources of concentrated omegas-3s and amino acid content. This not only works wonders for the muscles but also promotes heart health, brain health and improved immunity. And if you're not into spending $10 a pound on Wild Alaskan Salmon then that's not an issue; because eggs, chicken, nuts, red meat and Greek yogurt are other ideal options.

Just a quick tip: Please do not neglect or ignore the importance of eating fruits and vegetables on a daily basis. Healthy diets rich in fruits and veggies may reduce the risk of cancer and chronic diseases, while providing essential vitamins, minerals, fibers and other crucial substances, according to the Centers for Disease Control and Prevention. They may not seem essential to building muscle, but not pointing out their value to the body is nonsensical. Opt for buying organic fruits and veggies if possible.

Also, try not to load up on carbohydrates on non-training days. Many people make the dreadful mistake of consuming high-carb foods and drinks while inactive. And the end result? The excess amount of carbs is then stored in the body as fat. Spare your high-carb meals for breakfast and after workouts and avoid the common blunder of consuming exercise carbs on non-training days.

Summary: *Fish, chicken, turkey, nuts, eggs, quinoa, fruits and vegetables are all great examples of quality superfoods. Spread out your meals during the day and try to eat 4-6 small to medium meals throughout the day. Also, stop being obsessed with these low-fat diets. Healthy fats are essential for the human body and brain.*

Tip #3: Sleep, Sleep, Sleep

Sleep is essential for an individual's health and well-being. However, millions of individuals in the United States are absolutely unaware or disregard the fact that adequate sleep is crucial for maintaining a healthy lifestyle. I'm surprised at how many people seeking to build muscle are downright clueless about the importance of sleep on healthy muscle gain. Sleep dramatically affects the body's ability to repair damaged muscle tissue from serious training and helps replenish essential neurotransmitters that are crucial for a functional body. During sleep, your body maximizes its release of growth hormone, thus dramatically improving muscular recovery and development. "As your body enters into the non-REM deep sleep stage, your pituitary gland releases a shot of growth hormone that stimulates tissue growth and muscle repair. Growth hormone deficiency is associated with increased obesity, loss of muscle mass and reduced exercise capacity" states Becky Miller of the Livestrong Foundation.

Regardless of how hard you train your body during the day, without the proper amount of sleep, your body will have extreme difficulty repairing damaged muscle tissue that's crucial for muscle growth. Not only does a good night sleep accelerate the body's processes to build stronger muscles, but it is also helps reduce the chances of cardiovascular disease, stress-related problems and a lack of focus, attention and mental sharpness. This may not seem like a big deal to people who only care about building ripped muscles, but without an energized body and brain, good luck trying to Squat a heavy weight load. Bottom line, a good night's sleep will go a long way in helping you conquer your health and fitness goals.

So what exactly is a good night's sleep? Is it 6, 7, 8, 9 hours? In all honesty, there is no one specific universal answer to this question because everyone's individual sleep needs vary. Some people can go as little as six hours of sleep a night and still perform at their peak level while others can go as long as 9 to 10 hours a night. However, according to most studies, the ideal amount of sleep time needed per night for a healthy adult is around 7 to 8 hours. This is only a general guideline of what most healthy adults need in order to feel focused, alert and energized throughout the day. If you truly want to know how much sleep your own body needs, then I recommend taking a few consecutive nights paying close attention to your body and figuring out your sleep needs.

Summary: Getting a good night's sleep on a consistent basis will reward the body in so many ways. Whether it's maintaining a healthy mind, body and spirit, or aiding the muscle-building process, a good night's sleep will go a long way in helping you feel and energized, focused, and mentally and physically prepared the next day.

10 Tips to a Better Night's Sleep

Tip 1: Establish a regular sleep schedule. Try to go to a sleep around the same time every night.

Tip 2: Avoid the blue lights before bedtime. Televisions, computers, phones, etc. should be avoided at least a few hours prior to going to bed.

Tip 3: Alcohol, caffeine (tea, sodas, coffee) and cigarettes should be avoided since they make act like stimulants.

Tip 4: Avoid drinking excessive fluids near bedtime since that may cause you to wake up in the middle of the night.

Tip 5: Morning and afternoon exercise has been linked to getting a good night's sleep, however avoid vigorous exercise at least 4-6 hours before bedtime. Intense training acts like a stimulant and energizes the body and brain.

Tip 6: Avoid daytime naps.

Tip 7: Avoid facing the alarm clock toward you while on bed. This can cause you to feel anxious when trying to fall asleep.

Tip 8: Avoid watching any intense, dramatic or depressing movies, shows or videos while trying to sleep.

Tip 9: Make sure you're in a dark, quiet room with no distractors keeping you awake. Also make sure that the room temperature is best suited for you.

Tip 10: Avoid eating late and heavy meals before going to sleep. Opt for a light snack like a PB&J sandwich or Greek Yogurt.

Tip #4: Learn proper form & technique

One of the most disturbing parts of exercising in a crowded area is looking around and finding individuals perform exercises with bad technique and form. In certain cases, I feel an eager temptation to going up to the individual and informing him just how dreadful his technique really is. In other instances, I feel as if every other man occupying the Squat rack has his own special version of how to perform a Squat. I have witnessed some scary stuff in my years of weightlifting. Please, hear me out when I say that there's nothing more imperative when it comes to lifting weights then lifting with good form and technique. Taking the necessary time to read articles, watch free videos, join a workout session with a personal trainer, or practice the movement yourself will help ensure that you're not blindly lifting heavy weights improperly. Improper weight lifting techniques is the quickest way to sabotage your body's ability to grow lean muscle mass and experience great strength gains. For instance, if you're performing an exercise like the Squat incorrectly, then instead of the quads, hips and glutes being fully contracted in the movement; other muscle groups like the back or joints will be forced to carry the extra workload. This unnecessary tension and stress inflicted on these muscles could cause serious issues in the long run; especially with a heavy workload. No one wants to deal with potentially suffering from a muscle strain or ruptured disc in the low back due to incorrect form. This will not only induce a world of pain on the body, but will also cause minor or even serious problems long-term. Numerous risks and hazards are associated with incorrect weightlifting form. This is why it's crucial to learn the proper form and technique of different exercises.

Adding too much weight on the bar is another way to drastically influence the correctness of your form. Risking the precision of your technique in order to throw on another 10 pounds of weight is just not worth it. If there's one thing to remember from all this, it's that good form should be prioritized over weight use.

Secondly, make sure that you're listening to your body. If you're doing Dumbbell Shoulder Presses, then you should feel tension on your shoulders. Bicep Curls are intended to cause tension to the Biceps. There is nothing scientific about this. If you are somehow feeling tension in your middle or low back when performing Biceps Curls or Shoulder Presses, then you're obviously doing something wrong. Always make sure that you're feeling the contractions in the muscle and that the intended target muscle is doing all of the work. By getting off on the wrong foot, you'll decelerate the muscle growth process and cause potential tension and stress in undesirable places like the low back.

For those of you readers who want to see significant improvements in muscle mass, strength gains and muscle growth can rest assured that proper lifting form and technique will help accelerate these processes. The only exception to this is machine-based exercises because of how easy it is to perform the movement. Nonetheless, if you're more inclined to performing free weight exercises like the Squat, Deadlift and Bench Press, then it's imperative to learn and practice carrying out near-perfect form at a certain weight range before progressing to heavier workloads.

Summary: Correct form and technique throughout the entire movement is a key factor to getting the most out of your hard work. Prioritize the correctness of your form and always look for ways to improve your technique to further maximize the body's ability to build lean muscle. And if you need help, utilize the resources around you.

Tip #5: Focus on Compound Exercises

Most beginners who start out lifting weights are usually oblivious about recognizing the difference between compound and isolation exercises. Because most beginners don't know the difference, they spend more and more time literally walking from one exercise machine to the next until they've walked around the entire gym complex. I call them "nomads" because they literally wander from place to place in search for the next great machine. If you are serious about effectively and efficiently building lean muscle and gaining pure strength, then your primary focus and attention shall rely on performing compound exercises.

Compound exercises, in simple terms, are movements that target and train multiple muscles and joints in the body instead of just one. Prime examples of compound movements are Squats, Deadlifts, Bench Press, Military Press, Hang Cleans and Pull-Ups. These compound exercises not only train multiple muscles all at once, but they teach different muscle groups in the body to work together to carry out the movement. One prime example is the Squat, which trains and stabilizes the Quads, Hips, Glutes, Hamstrings, Low Back and abdominals. The reason that I throw in muscle groups like the low back and core is because while performing a Squat, the upper back, low back and abdominals are all being trained to coordinate the entire movement. By effectively training and stabilizing multiple muscle groups all in the form of a single movement, you're efficiently building muscle and strength in the entire body while burning fat. Performing movements such as the Squat will accelerate strength gains, muscle growth and fat burn.

Another plus about compound exercises like the Squat is that they dramatically improve communication between the brain and other muscle groups. Because exercises like the Squat incorporate several muscle groups to carry out the movement all together, it trains and teaches the muscle groups in the body to work together to coordinate and balance the movement. This may appear nonsensical, but in reality, compound exercises can go a long way in promoting not only gains in strength and size, but also in mobility, balance and coordination. But isolation exercises, i.e. most of the machines in the gym, like Leg Presses, Leg Curls and Leg Extensions don't possess the same benefits as compound exercises. That doesn't mean you should eliminate these exercises entirely. An isolation exercise like the Bicep Curl is probably the best exercise when it comes to building strength and size in the biceps. However, if you're seeking to accelerate growth and maximum gains in muscle-building while burning fat, then it's almost imperative that you test the power of compound exercises.

This also pertains to athletes who engage in sprinting, jumping and throwing. All of these movements require multiple muscle groups to activate and work together. Consequently, training your muscles to work together with compound exercises will boast your body's capability to carry out these movements at maximum efficiency.

In closing, just remember that compound exercises are first priority, isolation exercises come second.

Summary: *Focusing on compound exercises, instead of isolation exercises, will help build muscle and gain pure strength more effectively and efficiently. Don't neglect isolation exercises altogether, but remember that compound exercises should take first priority in your weightlifting routine.*

Tip #6: High Reps vs. Low Reps

There is ongoing debate between which type of exercise routine is best for muscle growth and development. Some say high reps with light weight is better for muscle development, while others strongly insist that performing low reps with heavy weight is ideal for muscle growth. By high repetitions I mean anywhere from 8-12 reps and for low repetitions anywhere between 1-5 reps. Olympic lifting and powerlifting athletes tend to focus more on the lower rep range because focusing on lifting heavier weight effectively facilitates the body for better strength gains. This is crucial for power lifters and Olympic trainees because they need to train to lift the heaviest amount of weight possible for competitions. On the other hand, bodybuilders commonly tend to focus on the higher rep range of 8-12 because this means that the body will go under an increase time under tension and stress. By further pushing your muscles to lift moderate weight under excessive tension, you're stimulating the flow of anabolic-hormone levels in the body, including the all-important growth hormone testosterone. This evidently leads to increases in muscular growth and definition, which is highly prioritized in the bodybuilding world.

However, while a routine characterized by high reps usually means more physique, spending too much time in this rep range makes it difficult to increase the weight. Evidently, this holds several disadvantages for someone looking to increase muscular strength. There is a huge disparity between someone who looks strong and someone who actually is strong. Though the higher rep approach promises muscular growth and size, it doesn't fulfill the promise of astounding gains in strength. If you were to look at the body composition of current Deadlift world-record holder Zydrunas Savickas, lifting a total of 1155 pounds in the 2014 Arnold Strongman Classic, you'll clearly notice that he doesn't necessarily have the flashiest muscles in the world. But he is one of the strongest men in the world, no doubt about it. This is why yet again, it is essential that you also spend some time in the low rep range if you're serious about developing strength and lifting more weight than you ever thought possible. By patiently spending time in the low rep range (1-5 reps per set) with near maximal weight, you are forcing your body to recruit more motor units and muscle fibers to facilitate the heavier lifting. This in turn will cause your strength gains to go beyond the roof, though your physique will appear nothing like those flashy bodybuilders.

Mike Robertson, C.S.C.S., recommends spending dedicated periods of time on each end of the spectrum. As Robertson states, "The general rule is to spend at least 4-6 weeks focusing on one end before you even think about heading to the other." That is, focusing on high reps with moderate weight for a reasonable period of time before switching off to more low-rep, heavy weight action. As long as you make the conscious effort of maintaining balance in your workout routine, you should experience remarkable progress in overall muscular strength, growth and definition.

Summary: *Though high rep sets (8-12 reps) fulfills muscle growth and size, don't neglect the importance of building strength with low-rep sets (1-5 sets). Implement both methods of training, 4-6 weeks on each end of the spectrum, to get the most out of your weightlifting routine.*

Tip #7: Post-Workout Protein

Any bodybuilder who obsesses over building as much muscle mass as possible already recognizes the importance of consuming post-workout protein. This is because post-workout liquid shakes helps weary muscles rebuild and recover after suffering a beating in the gym. When I say "rebuild and recover" I mean increasing skeletal muscle protein synthesis, increasing glycogen storage in the muscle, and consequently aiding bigger overall gains in strength and lean muscle mass. Probably the third most critical factor when it comes to building muscle is a protein-carb rich, well-balanced diet. Exercise and water, I believe, are the leading two. Consuming a post-workout protein drink after exercise is an integral part of any great muscle-building diet.

Though a post-workout meal may suffice in terms of helping the body recover from a workout session, almost every fitness source recommends drinking a protein-rich beverage so that the body could absorb it faster. John M. Berardi, one of the world's foremost experts in nutrition, explains it this way: "A liquid post-exercise formula may be fully absorbed within 30 to 60 minutes, providing much needed muscle nourishment by this time. However, a slower digesting solid food meal may take 2 to 3 hours to fully reach the muscle."

Now many of you might be saying to yourselves "Why does it matter how long it takes my body to absorb nutrients after exercise?" Well, timing makes all the difference considering the fact that your muscles are damaged, weary and fatigued after a brutal workout. Therefore, your muscles are immediately open to taking in nutrients that will begin and speed up the process of muscle recovery and growth. This is why many nutrition experts strongly insist that you consume an acceptable amount of protein immediately after completing your workout session. The Nutrition Coaching Company™ puts it this way "As soon as you drop that last dumbbell, you should be consuming some post workout nutrition."

Now here are the two critical questions: How many grams of protein should I aim for after exercise? Should I try to consume as much protein as possible after exercise? Based on what I've read from other Ph.D. level nutritionists, fitness experts and coaches, any recovery drink that consists of around 20 grams of protein is sufficient for proper muscle fiber production and protein synthesis. Case in point, 20 grams of protein is the "sweet spot" for building a lean muscle-building machine. Try to make a conscious effort to stay in between the 20-30 gram range for protein intake.

In regards to the misleading myth that the more protein you consume after exercise the better, I could confidently proclaim that that is false! Allow Russell Abaray and Douglas Boatwright of the National Strength and Conditioning Association (NSCA) to explain, "Many times, individuals taking protein supplements will ingest too many grams causing the nitrogen balance in the body to be thrown off. Subsequently, the excess protein is excreted in the urine. The ingestion of excess protein supplements may place additional stress on the kidneys and liver, and may result in dehydration, calcium loss, and gastrointestinal problems." So to answer the previous question: No! More protein does not equal better results.

Summary: Always consume an immediate source of protein after intense training. A post-workout protein beverage, i.e. protein shakes or chocolate milk should be prioritized over regular meals because it's absorbed quickly to nourish weary, tired muscles. Aim for 20 to 25 grams of protein after intense training.

Tip #8: Protein Supplements vs. Chocolate Milk

Earlier in this book I explained the underlying benefits of drinking a good post-workout beverage immediately after exercise. Anyone who's shopped in the past decade is probably aware of the hundreds of protein supplements invading the aisles of top supermarkets. Whether its Protein bars, shakes, powders, pills, or other things of that nature; individuals looking to gain muscle mass have been bombarded with tons of factory-made products promising to transform them into bodybuilding gods. Though these supplements do help pack on pounds of muscle, most of them are highly-priced and others are even unsafe to use. What many of us fail to realize is that there are other natural and inexpensive solutions to getting quality, high-value protein.

Studies have shown that low-fat chocolate milk has been scientifically proven to be one of the best post-workout recovery drinks for rebuilding, refueling and reshaping the muscles. Some studies even go as far as to label it as the ideal post-workout drink because of its natural source of high quality protein, ideal 3-1 carb-protein ratio and essential fluids and electrolytes; i.e. sodium, potassium, calcium and magnesium. The 3-1 carbohydrate-to-protein ratio is a key factor because it is the ideal carb-to-protein ratio for optimal skeletal muscle protein synthesis and net muscle protein balance. The natural, high-quality source of protein content and essential fluids and electrolytes are also beneficial for strength gains, improved muscle mass and fat loss. Not to mention that the fact that it is both inexpensive and available almost everywhere.

Personally, I prefer chocolate milk as my post-workout recovery drink over popular protein shakes and powders. But bodybuilders tend to go with protein supplements. Most bodybuilders know that protein supplements like whey and casein powders are excellent options for maximum strength gains, body mass, body shape and muscle growth.

However, I cannot fully vouch for all the great benefits of supplements considering the fact that I do not take them. I have also read certain publications that reveal some alarming truths about protein supplements. Maybe in another book I'll breakdown the "secret hazardous effects of protein supplements that health companies may not be telling you."

The only thing that I could suggest about supplement use is to avoid consuming excessive dose amounts, because like I said earlier, this could lead to future problems in the kidneys and liver. Always aim for about 20-25 grams, or 1 scoop of protein powder after workouts.

One interesting fact to point out is that under the Dietary Supplement Health and Education Act of 1994 (DSHEA), protein supplements, like any other supplements, are not regulated by the FDA. Unfortunately for consumers, this means that supplements can be highly susceptible to concentrations of contaminants and pollutants; i.e. lead, cadmium, mercury, and arsenic. So make sure that you're not blindly something that could ultimately be destroying you. Always use common sense, do your research and look at the ingredients of popular supplement brands before consuming them. You'll never know what you might find out.

Summary: *Chocolate milk has been studies and proven to be an excellent source of muscle nourishment after a grueling task in the weight room. If you're tired of spending a fortune on protein powder and other supplements, then look no further. However, if you're into the idea that protein supplements are the way to go to build lean muscle, then more power to you. Just don't overdose and please read the ingredients label.*

Tip #9: Post-workout recovery techniques

Recovery after intense training is a prominent component for muscle repair and growth. One of the more popular but certainly not more effective ways to promote the recovery process after intense training is some form of static stretching. Static stretching is defined as a stretch held for a period of time while the body is at rest. I believe that static stretching is an effective method to lengthen tight muscles and improve range of motion. However, there has been little to no justification on whether static stretching is indeed beneficial to aiding the relief of muscle soreness after training. Interestingly, some doctors even claim that stretching actually decreases blood flow. This statement is noteworthy considering the fact that increases in blood circulation is a key factor to effectively repairing damaged tissues and muscles. So, in contrast to widely held beliefs, serious stretching after workout may be contraindicated for recovery. That does not mean avoid static stretches entirely. It just means that static stretching is not the most reliable method of aiding post-workout recovery.

Furthermore, I believe there are more effective ways to help weary muscles recover more efficiently. My suggestion is to start implementing other methods of recovery such as foam rolling or hydrotherapy. Foam rolling is a self-myofascial release (SMR) technique to inhibit overactive muscles. A foam roller is a powerful therapeutic tool that works as deep-tissue massage instrument to really ease the muscle tension and pain caused by intense exercise. Foam rolling promotes improved blood circulation in many areas in the body, lengthening of short muscles and optimal spinal range of motion. Certain studies not only support the legitimacy of foam rolling on repairing damaged muscles after exercise, but for also maintaining optimal health and well-being. I strongly recommend utilizing a foam roller not only for accelerating the recovery process but also for sustaining muscle tissue health. To foam roll properly, apply moderate pressure to a specific muscle or muscle group using your bodyweight. Roll gently along the tight muscle area until you have reached the joints, and slowly roll back up. Do not roll on or past the joints! If used properly, this therapeutic tool will serve immediate effects on muscle recovery and restoration.

Other notable methods of reducing muscle aches and fatigue after exercise are ice baths, cold showering and hydrotherapy. Hydrotherapy, in simple terms, is a therapeutic technique that combines the use of hot water and cold water to relieve discomfort and promote well-being. A great example of practicing hydrotherapy is taking a very hot shower for 2 minutes, followed by 30 seconds of cold water, and then back-and-forth repeatedly for at least 3 times. This is an extremely effective method of easing the muscle pain and soreness after intense physical activity. You can either utilize this method of aiding recovery or opt for an ice bath or cold shower.

Whether it's the practice of foam rolling, hydrotherapy, ice baths or just taking a cold shower; find a recovery plan that's best suitable for you.

Summary: Taking a cold shower, an ice bath, foam rolling, or practicing hydrotherapy are just some alternative ways to recover quicker from intense training. Static stretching, though ideal for increasing range of motion, is simply not that effective to helping repair damaged, weary muscles. Help ease muscle pain and soreness with an alternative method.

Tip #10: Warm-Up before Training

Before even considering putting on your weight-lifting belt and beginning to squat tons of weight; don't forget the importance of warming up for at least 5-10 minutes. A good warm-up before weightlifting serves many purposes for the body like inducing an increase in temperature and blood flow, loosening the joints and muscles for physical activity and reducing the risk of injury. The increase in blood flow to the brain stimulates mental focus, sharpness and energy. This will go a long way on the days you feel sluggish and lazy. Some great methods of effectively preparing the body are light cardio, dynamic stretching and "warm-up" repetitions. I recommend incorporating all three if possible. A light cardio of 5 minutes on the treadmill or stationary bicycle, followed by dynamic stretches like arm swings, lunges, windmills and such, and a quick warm-up set or two is a great example of a warm-up. A warm up like this helps get the blood flowing and temperatures rising before starting the strength training session.

There are many ways to go about this, and feel free to mix and match any combination of movements that you like. If you are an athlete who competes in football, basketball, baseball or any other sport, then I recommend performing speed and agility drills related to your sport before weightlifting. There are many young athletes who will benefit greatly from spending 5-10 minutes practicing speed drills as a quick warm-up. Jumping rope is yet another great way to wake up the muscles and is suitable for both athletes and regular individuals. I personally spend 5 minutes just doing random drills because to wake up my body before intense physical activity. The point is that a good warm-up should get your heart pumping, blood flowing and body sweating. That does not mean that you should start doing cardio training before strength training. That is actually the opposite of what most fitness experts and coaches recommend for active individuals. By making the dreadful mistake of doing cardiovascular training before strength training, you will dramatically deplete the amount of energy required to perform intense strength training. Lower energy levels in the body equals lower intensity, focus and efficiency to lift heavy weight. And the lower the intensity, the less production there is; leading to slower gains in muscle strength, mass and growth.

Now on the opposite spectrum, if you are more inclined toward increasing cardiovascular endurance, then doing cardio training prior to strength training is probably a better option. But if you're primary focus is gaining lean muscle mass and strength like most people reading this book, then the best option is sticking to doing strength training prior to cardiovascular training.

Now, just to clarify, I'm not suggesting or endorsing the fact that you must perform cardio training after strength training. Performing intense cardio is definitely not a prerequisite that needs to be fulfilled in order to relinquish the maximum benefits of consistent strength training. However, if you're seeking to maximize the body's ability to eliminate fat, then a round of cardio training after strength training will help assist that process.

In closing, warming up for 5-10 minutes before physical activity is an essential aspect of your weightlifting routine.

Summary: *A 5-10 minute warm-up will better prepare the body and muscles for physical intensity. Do not overlook the significance of properly warming up the body before pushing, pulling and lifting heavy weight. Athletes can perform speed and agility drills related to their sport, and individuals can jump rope or run on a treadmill to warm-up the body.*

Tip #11: Add Variety to your Workouts

Anyone who possesses a true desire of achieving incredible gains in muscular strength has probably done endless research on discovering the best exercises for muscle strength and mass. No doubt, I am definitely one of those people who repeatedly attempted to discover the ground-breaking, super-efficient exercises for acquiring supernatural strength. But what I had failed to realize in my pursuit of muscle-building wisdom was that limiting my body to only a few exercises would not benefit me in the long run. This is because when it comes to exercising the body, change is good.

For example, there are many beginners out there who assume that the best way to increase overall chest strength is to rely solely on performing the Bench Press. Though the Bench Press is probably the leading exercises for building chest strength, individuals seeking to train their chest to its greatest potential should not neglect other chest-strengthening exercises. The Incline Bench Press, Decline Bench Press, DB* Press, DB* Flies, Wide-Grip Bench Press, Push-Up, and Cable Press are all great options for overall chest strength. The traditional Bench Press does not effectively incorporate the muscles in the upper chest and lower chest. Have you ever struggled mightily on lifting a lightly-weighted bar on an Incline Bench? If so, it's probably due to the lack of strength in the upper chest area. By not properly training other areas of the chest with other exercises, consequently, you will set yourself up for stagnation and the all-to-common "bench plateau."

This truth does not only apply to the chest, but to any major muscle group in the body; i.e. Quads, Hamstrings, Shoulders and Biceps. Bottom line, to reach your body's maximum potential for strength, size and definition, it's critical that you incorporate a variety of movements in your workout routine. Variations of the Squat include the Front Squat, Pause Squat and the Bulgarian Split Squat.

You can also perform Lunges, Leg Press and Step-Ups for quadriceps strength. There are many ways you mix and match different movements into your workout routine, but never remain content with sticking to the same workout script. A routine characterized by "sameness" will result in boredom, stagnation and lack of progression.

Summary: Change is good, when it comes to weightlifting. Never settle with doing the same exercises over and over again. Mix and match a variety of exercises in your physical training routine to obtain better gains in strength, size and muscle growth over time.

* Dumbbell

Tip #12: Spread the Workload, Don't Neglect Any Muscle Group

When it comes to weightlifting, most individuals tend to value certain exercises over others. Almost every veteran power lifter or bodybuilder has an all-time favorite exercise that they treasure more than any other exercise out there. There is certainly no crime against having your own preferred exercise to perform. However, it's an offense to the body when you start neglecting certain muscle groups altogether in your workout routine. By entirely abandoning certain major muscle groups, you'll not only sabotage the body's ability to possess strength and muscle, but this blunder will also result in heavy muscular imbalances.

Human movement and function requires a balance of muscle length and strength between opposing muscles surrounding a joint, according to Dr. Vladimir Janda. Muscle imbalance occurs when one side of the opposing muscles is excessively stronger than the other. For example, the biceps and triceps are two muscle groups that perform opposite motions. If the triceps are substantially weak to the point where it's not capable of balancing the force applied by much stronger biceps, then that's a muscular imbalance.

The major muscle groups work in pairs to carry out different functions in the body. The biceps and triceps work together to bend and straighten the elbow. The quadriceps and hamstrings work together to bend and straighten the knee. By balancing out the workload on each major muscle group when weightlifting, you'll help prevent serious muscular imbalances in the elbows and knees. Consequently, it is critical to spread the load among the major muscle groups in the body to maximize your muscle growth potential.

Furthermore, if you're looking to gain bigger arms, then it's important to note that the human arm is primarily comprised of triceps and not the biceps.

So if you think that performing endless sets of Bicep Curls and neglecting triceps exercises is beneficial to getting bigger arms, then you're wrong. Do not make the dreadful mistake of consistently training the same muscle group without training the opposite muscle group. If you are obsessed with performing Back Squats, then that's okay as long as you're maintaining some form of balance with hamstring-strengthening exercises like the Deadlift.

In closing, target the whole body with movements that help strengthen each muscle group in the body. Maintaining muscular balance is a key aspect of weightlifting that is overlooked by many. Don't repeat the same error that many others make, but spread the workload among the entire body for maximum growth.

Summary: *Intense training on the Biceps without any Triceps-strengthening exercise is a recipe for disaster. If you want lean muscle mass and strength throughout the entire body, then learn to train the entire body. It's that simple.*

Tip #13: Warning: Avoid Overtraining

Although exercise is important for a variety of reasons like health, a longer lifespan, vitality, strength, energy and self-confidence; it's also very important that you're not overstating your welcome in the gym. By spending hours on end pushing, pulling and lifting heavy loads of weight without proper recovery, at some point you will physically exhaust the body enough to sabotage your fitness goals. One of the most common mistakes many beginners make is overtraining the muscles. Overtraining occurs when you repeatedly train your body to the point that you've exceeded your body's recovery capacity. In short, either the training itself was too extreme or your recovery time between workouts was too short.

There are many dangers and risks involved in overtraining the body. Some of these risks include increased chances of injury, pain in muscles and joints, sudden drop in performance (for athletes) and decreases in strength. I can't begin to explain the importance of avoiding exercise burnout and providing adequate rest and recovery for the body between sessions. I figured this out the hard way, when I participated in Outdoor Track & Field in high school. I had high expectations going into my third and final season, and I had spent hours and hours in the gym every other night doing the best I could to physically prepare myself. Ironically however, it turns out that my muscles were exhausted to the point where my performance actually declined significantly. Instead of everything coming together as I expected, quite the opposite happened due to the fact that I overtrained. Consequently, I ended up running some of the worst times in the 400 and 800 meter dashes that year. Obviously, that was not to best way to finish off my running career. I should have listened to the advice of a dear friend of mine who told me "Hard work does not equal progress."

Do the best you can to avoid overtraining your muscles. Keep your workout sessions at a maximum of around 60 minutes and make sure you are giving your body sufficient time to recuperate. For example, if you're planning on training the whole body on Monday, then I recommended taking at least a day off before the next session. Giving your body the recovery and rest it needs on Tuesday will help ensure that you are not overtraining the muscles. The vast majority of strength and conditioning experts recommend limiting your workout sessions between 45 and 60 minutes and giving yourself somewhere between 24-48 hours to recover from training. The reason behind this logic has to do with a hormone in the body called cortisol. Cortisol is a hormone produced in the cortex of the adrenal gland and is triggered in response to stress. As you might know, constantly lifting, pushing and pulling heavy weight puts the muscles under heavy amounts of tension and stress. Training the body for too long or for too high of an intensity will cause cortisol levels to spike rapidly. As cortisol levels begin to elevate to all-time highs, total testosterone concentrations begin to decline. When this starts to happen, workouts then become counterproductive to your goals. This simple visual demonstration of the relationship between cortisol and testosterone is worth a thousand words:

$$\uparrow \text{Cortisol} = \downarrow \text{Testosterone}$$

Therefore, it is imperative that you minimize your workout sessions to around 60 minutes and give your body the necessary rest and recovery time it needs to do it again.

In closing, remember that more work does not always equal progress in the gym. Arrive at the gym with a focused attitude and never overstate your welcome.

Summary: Do not overtrain; period. If you're doing whole-body workouts then give yourself at least a day's rest in-between workout sessions for adequate recovery. Regardless of what training method you use, make sure that you're not targeting the same muscle group on consecutive days.

Tip #14: The Power of Supersets

A great way to build muscle while burning serious fat is executing an advanced training method known as supersets. However, before I advance any further, let me proclaim that this is advanced technique is not always recommended for beginner weightlifters. The reason being is because supersets are very intense and challenging, especially for newcomers. Sticking to basic weight lifting principles as a beginner is highly recommended to build a strong foundation of strength before shifting to more intense techniques. Some experts recommend having at least six months to a year under your belt before incorporating more advanced training styles such as this one.

However, there is no need to withhold this information from readers who could potentially benefit from this advice in the near future. So I am going to briefly discuss the benefits of Supersets, what they are, and how to effectively include this training technique into your routine. A Superset, otherwise known as a "combined set," is an advanced technique that combines two or more exercises together to increase efficiency and workload in a shorter span of time. A great example of a superset is a workout that alternates between the Bench Press and Push-Ups. For instance, an individual performs a set of Bench Presses, followed by Push-Ups, then back to Bench Presses, then Push-Ups, and so on. This technique is a great way to elevate the intensity level and burn fat by increasing the heart rate level. Other examples of supersets are Close-Grip Bench Presses paired with Chin-Ups, Lunges with Single-Leg Deadlifts, Bicep Curls with Dips, Front Raises with Lateral Raises, etc. The benefits of performing supersets is that they save time, increase efficiency, maximize intensity and effectively work your muscles.

What's interesting about supersets is the fact that you're able to freely mix and match any two exercises you want. This makes supersets more convenient and flexible to utilize.

Supersets that combine two exercises that train opposing muscle groups are the best options in my opinion. Let me distinguish the difference between supersets that target one muscle group and supersets that target opposing muscle groups. Supersets that target the same muscle group are Dips with Triceps Extensions, Bench Press with Push-Ups, Leg Press with Squats, etc. As you may realize, these supersets are more focused on brutally training the same muscle group. On the other hand, supersets that target two or more muscle groups are, like I said before, Bicep Curls with Dips, Squats with Hamstring Curls, Bench Presses with Pull-Ups and things of that nature. These supersets are more inclined to training multiple and opposing muscle groups for maximum efficiency.

I always recommend performing supersets that work one muscle followed by the opposing muscle. Just imagine doing Bench Presses-Push-Ups as a superset followed by Incline Bench Presses-Dumbbell Press as another. A workout of that nature would leave the chest muscles impaired for days. In my opinion, the safest way to incorporate Supersets into your routine is to train opposing muscle groups or different but non-opposing muscle groups. This will not only save a ton of time in the gym but also help promote fat loss and muscular balance in the body.

In closing, remember that training technique is not recommended for beginners who have not built a strong foundation of strength. Spend at least 3 months building a foundation of strength and muscle before progressing to more advanced training techniques.

Summary: Supersets are great for intensifying workouts, saving time and maximizing exercise productivity. If you really want to burn fat while weightlifting, then performing supersets will help get the job done. However, this is an advanced training technique and is not recommended for beginners.

Final Thoughts

I would like to thank you, the reader, for taking the time to read this book and gain helpful insights about improving your health. Remember that the decisions you make outside the gym are just as crucial to building muscle as the decisions you make inside the gym. Also, keep in mind that though these tips are useful, there is an even greater significance of possessing the right mentality. Persistency, confidence, motivation, toughness, and integrity are all key components to maintaining an effective weightlifting routine. Be strong to get strong. Grow up to grow muscle. Get big to get bigger. And most importantly, have fun with it.

Best Regards

www.ingramcontent.com/pod-product-compliance
Lightning Source LLC
Chambersburg PA
CBHW020401290526
45785CB00005B/2386